Fibromyalgia

Complete Guide to Understanding, Diagnosing, and Managing Fibromyalgia, Chronic Pain, Fatigue, and Effective Symptom Relief Strategies

Graham Julian Oliver

Disclaimer

The information contained in this book, *Fibromyalgia: Complete Guide to Understanding, Diagnosing, and Managing Fibromyalgia, Chronic Pain, Fatigue, and Effective Symptom Relief Strategies*, is for educational and informational purposes only. It is not intended to be a substitute for professional medical advice, diagnosis, or treatment. Always seek the advice of your physician or other qualified health provider with any questions you may have regarding a medical condition or treatment.

The author and publisher do not guarantee the accuracy, completeness, or usefulness of any information contained in this book. The information may not apply to every individual or situation, and reliance on any information provided in this book is solely at your own risk.

The author does not endorse any individual, product, website, organization, or other names that may be referenced or mentioned within this book. All such references are made solely for informational purposes and should not be construed as endorsements.

In no event shall the author or publisher be liable for any direct, indirect, incidental, special, consequential, or punitive damages arising out of or in connection with the use of this book or the information provided herein.

By reading this book, you acknowledge that you have read this disclaimer and agree to its terms.

About This Book

The book *Fibromyalgia: Complete Guide to Understanding, Diagnosing, and Managing Fibromyalgia, Chronic Pain, Fatigue, and Effective Symptom Relief Strategies* serves as a vital resource for individuals grappling with the multifaceted nature of fibromyalgia. This comprehensive guide not only defines and explores the complexities of fibromyalgia but also addresses the wide array of symptoms that can disrupt daily life. By providing a thorough understanding of the condition, readers can appreciate the significance of early diagnosis and the critical role it plays in managing symptoms effectively. Furthermore, the text emphasizes the importance of recognizing fibromyalgia's unique characteristics, distinguishing it from other chronic pain conditions while unpacking the neurobiological factors involved.

Additionally, the guide underscores the necessity of personalized management plans, encouraging readers to take an active role in their health journey. It delves into the expected challenges and adjustments that may arise, providing a roadmap to navigate lifestyle changes that can alleviate symptoms. With an emphasis on identifying personal triggers, the guide equips readers with strategies for managing their condition, creating an environment conducive to symptom relief. Moreover, it highlights the importance of support networks and available resources, ensuring that individuals feel connected and empowered throughout their journey.

The book also tackles the symptoms and diagnostic process with clarity, guiding readers through common symptoms and the importance of maintaining detailed symptom journals for effective communication with healthcare providers. By demystifying the diagnostic challenges often faced by fibromyalgia patients, it encourages advocacy and open dialogue with medical professionals. Furthermore, the exploration of potential causes and triggers—ranging from genetics to environmental factors—provides a holistic view of the condition, fostering understanding and compassion towards one's experiences.

In addressing symptom management, the guide offers an array of self-management strategies, incorporating alternative therapies, dietary adjustments, and lifestyle modifications that can significantly enhance well-being. The focus on holistic approaches ensures that readers not only learn about conventional medical treatments but also discover valuable insights into integrating alternative therapies into their daily routines. The emphasis on lifestyle modifications, including the significance of a balanced diet and stress management techniques, helps readers cultivate healthier habits that support long-term health.

A significant section dedicated to coping with fatigue addresses one of the most debilitating aspects of fibromyalgia, equipping readers with strategies for managing energy levels and maintaining productivity. This focus on practical solutions empowers individuals to establish a balanced daily schedule and recognize the importance of rest, creating a framework for better management of both physical and mental fatigue.

Support systems are a central theme of the book, emphasizing the importance of community and communication. The guide provides actionable advice on building a robust support network, ensuring that individuals with fibromyalgia can share their experiences and access the emotional support necessary for navigating their journey. Furthermore, it encourages self-advocacy and education for loved ones, fostering understanding and strengthening relationships.

Finally, the guide offers inspiration through personal stories and reflections, motivating readers to embrace life with fibromyalgia. By celebrating progress and resilience, this book not only serves as a practical manual but also as a source of encouragement for individuals seeking to live fulfilling lives despite the challenges posed by fibromyalgia. Through its comprehensive approach, the guide stands as a beacon of hope and empowerment for all those impacted by this condition.

Table of Contents

Introduction

Definition and Overview of Fibromyalgia

Fibromyalgia is a chronic disorder characterized by widespread musculoskeletal pain, fatigue, and tenderness in localized areas. It affects how the brain processes pain signals, leading to heightened sensitivity to pain. While the exact cause of fibromyalgia remains unclear, it is believed to involve a combination of genetic, environmental, and psychological factors. Understanding this condition is crucial for effective management, as it affects both physical and emotional well-being.

The prevalence of fibromyalgia is significant, impacting millions of people worldwide, predominantly women. It is often associated with other conditions, such as anxiety, depression, and irritable bowel syndrome. Awareness of fibromyalgia's unique challenges helps patients recognize their symptoms and seek appropriate medical attention, paving the way for effective treatment and support.

Common Symptoms and Their Impact on Daily Life

Common symptoms of fibromyalgia include widespread pain, fatigue, sleep disturbances, and cognitive difficulties, often referred to as "fibro fog." Patients may experience muscle stiffness, headaches, and irritable bowel syndrome, contributing to an overall decline in quality of life. These symptoms can fluctuate, making daily activities challenging, as individuals may find it difficult to maintain a regular work schedule, engage in social activities, or perform household tasks.

The impact of these symptoms extends beyond physical discomfort; they can lead to emotional distress, affecting relationships and mental health. Patients often struggle with feelings of isolation, frustration, and uncertainty, making it essential to address both physical and emotional aspects of fibromyalgia in any management plan.

The Importance of Early Diagnosis and Management

Early diagnosis of fibromyalgia is crucial for effective management and improving quality of life. Recognizing the symptoms and differentiating them from other conditions can help patients receive timely treatment, reducing the severity and duration of symptoms. Healthcare professionals may use specific criteria, including patient history and symptom evaluation, to diagnose fibromyalgia, often involving a process of elimination for other potential causes of pain.

Prompt management strategies can include medications, physical therapy, and lifestyle changes. Early intervention not only alleviates symptoms but also helps prevent complications such as anxiety and depression, empowering patients to regain control over their lives and pursue meaningful activities.

Brief Discussion on the Complexity of Fibromyalgia

Fibromyalgia is a complex condition with multifaceted origins, making it challenging to diagnose and treat. Its symptoms can vary widely between individuals, with some experiencing mild discomfort while others suffer debilitating pain. The interplay between genetics, neurobiology, and psychosocial factors complicates the understanding of fibromyalgia, highlighting the need for a personalized approach to treatment.

Moreover, the stigma surrounding fibromyalgia often leads to misunderstanding and misdiagnosis. Educating patients, families, and healthcare providers about the complexities of this condition can foster empathy and support, creating an environment conducive to healing and effective management.

Overview of Treatment Options and Self-Management Strategies

Treatment options for fibromyalgia typically involve a multidisciplinary approach that may include medications, physical therapy, and alternative therapies. Common medications include pain relievers, antidepressants, and anti-seizure drugs, tailored to each patient's specific symptoms. Physical therapy can enhance strength and flexibility, while alternative therapies such as acupuncture, yoga, and massage therapy may provide additional relief.

Self-management strategies are equally essential in managing fibromyalgia. Patients can benefit from adopting healthy lifestyle habits, including regular exercise, balanced nutrition, and stress management techniques such as mindfulness and meditation. Keeping a symptom diary can also help identify triggers and patterns, enabling patients to make informed decisions about their health and daily routines.

What to Expect in This Guide

This guide serves as a comprehensive resource for understanding fibromyalgia, chronic pain, and fatigue. You will learn about the symptoms, diagnostic criteria, and effective management strategies tailored to individual needs. Each section provides practical information that can help you navigate your journey with fibromyalgia and enhance your quality of life.

In addition to medical insights, the guide emphasizes self-advocacy and informed decision-making. Expect to find actionable steps, such as keeping a symptom diary, tracking triggers, and exploring various treatment options. This structured approach aims to empower you with knowledge and skills to effectively manage your condition.

Emphasis on the Importance of Personalized Management Plans

Creating a personalized management plan is essential for managing fibromyalgia effectively. This plan should consider your unique symptoms, lifestyle, and preferences, allowing for adjustments as needed. Begin by consulting with healthcare professionals who specialize in fibromyalgia to develop a tailored strategy that includes medications, therapies, and lifestyle changes.

Regularly reviewing and updating your management plan is crucial. Document your progress and any changes in symptoms, as this information can help you and your healthcare provider fine-tune your approach. Engaging in open communication about what works and what doesn't can significantly enhance your overall treatment experience.

Encouragement to Actively Participate in One's Own Health

Taking an active role in your health is vital when managing fibromyalgia. Start by educating yourself about the condition, treatments, and coping strategies. This knowledge enables you to make informed choices about your health and treatment options. Attend workshops, support groups, or online forums to connect with others who share similar experiences.

Incorporating self-care practices into your daily routine can also enhance your well-being. Simple activities like mindfulness, meditation, and gentle exercise, such as yoga or walking, can positively impact your mental and physical health. Remember, your active participation is crucial in navigating your health journey and finding effective relief strategies.

Understanding the Role of Lifestyle Changes in Symptom Management

Lifestyle changes play a significant role in managing fibromyalgia symptoms. Start by focusing on regular exercise, as it can help reduce pain and improve energy levels. Consider low-impact activities, such as swimming or cycling, which are less likely to exacerbate pain. Gradually increasing your activity level can help build endurance without overwhelming your body.

Nutrition is another critical aspect of symptom management. Aim for a balanced diet rich in whole foods, fruits, vegetables, lean proteins, and healthy fats. Staying hydrated and avoiding processed foods or excessive sugar can contribute to overall well-being. Keep track of how different foods affect your symptoms and adjust your diet accordingly.

Support and Resources Available Throughout the Journey

Support and resources are essential for anyone managing fibromyalgia. Start by seeking out local or online support groups where you can share experiences, gain insights, and learn from others facing similar challenges. These communities can provide emotional support and practical advice that can help you feel less isolated in your journey.

Additionally, various resources, including educational materials, webinars, and health professionals specializing in fibromyalgia, are available. Don't hesitate to explore these resources to gain more knowledge and skills for managing your condition.

CHAPTER 1:

What is Fibromyalgia?

Definition and Medical Classification of Fibromyalgia

Fibromyalgia is a chronic pain condition characterized by widespread musculoskeletal pain, fatigue, sleep disturbances, and cognitive issues, often referred to as "fibro fog." It is classified as a central pain syndrome, where the nervous system amplifies pain signals, leading to heightened sensitivity. To be diagnosed, patients typically experience pain in at least 11 of 18 designated tender points across the body for a minimum of three months.

Medical classification recognizes fibromyalgia under various systems, including the International Classification of Diseases (ICD) and the Diagnostic and Statistical Manual of Mental Disorders (DSM-5). The ICD categorizes it as a disease, while the DSM-5 acknowledges its psychosocial impact, highlighting the need for a comprehensive approach to treatment that includes both physical and mental health considerations.

Overview of How Fibromyalgia Differs from Other Chronic Pain Conditions

Fibromyalgia is distinct from other chronic pain conditions like arthritis or back pain in that it primarily affects the soft tissues rather than the joints or muscles directly. While arthritis is characterized by inflammation and joint damage, fibromyalgia involves a heightened response to pain stimuli without clear physical damage. This can lead to confusion during diagnosis, as standard imaging tests may not show any abnormalities.

Additionally, fibromyalgia is often accompanied by a range of symptoms beyond pain, such as fatigue, sleep disturbances, and cognitive difficulties. This multi-faceted nature sets it apart from other conditions, emphasizing the need for a holistic approach to managing symptoms through lifestyle changes, medication, and alternative therapies.

Explanation of the Neurobiological Factors Involved

Neurobiological factors play a crucial role in fibromyalgia, primarily through dysfunction in how the brain and spinal cord process pain signals. Research suggests that individuals with fibromyalgia may have alterations in neurotransmitter levels, such as serotonin and norepinephrine, which can affect mood and pain perception. This imbalance may lead to a heightened sensitivity to pain and other stimuli.

Moreover, neuroimaging studies have shown that the brains of those with fibromyalgia respond differently to pain compared to healthy individuals. They may exhibit increased activity in pain-related areas, contributing to the chronic pain experience. Understanding these neurobiological aspects can guide treatment options, focusing on medications that target neurotransmitter imbalances and therapies aimed at retraining the nervous system's response to pain.

Common Misconceptions about Fibromyalgia

Misconceptions about fibromyalgia often stem from a lack of understanding of the condition. One common belief is that fibromyalgia is not a "real" illness, which can lead to skepticism from both the public and medical professionals. This misconception can further stigmatize those with the condition, making them feel invalidated and unsupported in their struggles.

Another prevalent myth is that fibromyalgia is solely caused by psychological factors. While stress and emotional well-being can influence symptoms, fibromyalgia is a complex condition with biological, psychological, and environmental components. Recognizing the legitimacy of fibromyalgia as a multifaceted disorder is crucial for fostering empathy and understanding.

Statistics on Prevalence and Demographics

Fibromyalgia affects approximately 2-4% of the global population, with a significant prevalence among women, who are diagnosed at a rate of about 7 to 9 times higher than men. It can occur in all age groups but is most commonly diagnosed in middle-aged adults. Studies indicate that fibromyalgia is often under diagnosed, especially in men and minority populations, leading to a lack of awareness and resources for these groups.

Demographic data reveal that fibromyalgia is not limited to any specific ethnic or cultural background, but its impact varies across populations. Awareness of these statistics is essential for healthcare providers to recognize and address fibromyalgia in diverse patient populations, ensuring equitable access to treatment and support.

The Role of Genetics in Fibromyalgia

Genetics can significantly influence the development of fibromyalgia, with studies indicating that it tends to run in families. Certain genetic variations may predispose individuals to chronic pain conditions, including fibromyalgia. Understanding one's family history of fibromyalgia or related chronic pain disorders can provide insight into the potential risk of developing the condition.

Moreover, research is ongoing to identify specific genes linked to fibromyalgia symptoms, such as pain sensitivity and sleep disturbances. Genetic testing and counseling may become valuable tools for individuals at risk, helping them to manage their health proactively through lifestyle changes and early interventions.

How Fibromyalgia Affects Different Age Groups

Fibromyalgia can impact individuals across all age groups, but its presentation and challenges may vary. In children and adolescents, fibromyalgia symptoms can manifest as chronic fatigue, abdominal pain, and sleep disturbances, often leading to missed school days and social difficulties. Early recognition and intervention are crucial for managing symptoms and improving the quality of life in younger individuals.

In older adults, fibromyalgia symptoms may be compounded by age-related health issues, such as arthritis or osteoporosis. This can make diagnosis and treatment more complex, as overlapping conditions can mask fibromyalgia symptoms. Comprehensive assessments that consider the full range of an individual's health status are essential for developing effective management strategies for older adults with fibromyalgia.

Overview of Comorbid Conditions Associated with Fibromyalgia

Individuals with fibromyalgia frequently experience comorbid conditions, including chronic fatigue syndrome, irritable bowel syndrome (IBS), depression, and anxiety disorders. These comorbidities can exacerbate fibromyalgia symptoms, making it more challenging to manage the condition effectively. Understanding these associations can help healthcare providers tailor treatment plans to address both fibromyalgia and any accompanying conditions.

Managing comorbid conditions often requires a multi-faceted approach that incorporates lifestyle changes, medication, and therapy. For example, addressing anxiety and depression through cognitive-behavioral therapy (CBT) can improve pain management and overall well-being in individuals with fibromyalgia. Collaborative care among healthcare providers is vital to ensure a holistic treatment strategy.

Impact on Physical and Mental Health

Fibromyalgia significantly affects both physical and mental health. Physically, individuals may experience debilitating pain, fatigue, and sleep disturbances, leading to a decrease in physical activity and overall fitness. This lack of activity can further exacerbate pain and fatigue, creating a vicious cycle that is challenging to break.

Mentally, the chronic nature of fibromyalgia can lead to feelings of isolation, anxiety, and depression. The unpredictability of symptoms can make it difficult to maintain relationships and engage in social activities, compounding mental health challenges. Support networks, including therapy and support groups, can play a crucial role in helping individuals manage both physical and mental health impacts.

Discussion on the Stigma Surrounding Fibromyalgia

Stigma surrounding fibromyalgia often stems from misunderstandings about the condition and its symptoms. Many individuals face skepticism from healthcare providers and peers, leading to feelings of isolation and frustration. This stigma can discourage individuals from seeking help and can undermine their experiences and struggles with chronic pain.

Addressing stigma requires increased awareness and education about fibromyalgia among the general public and healthcare professionals. Advocacy for better understanding and acceptance can empower individuals with fibromyalgia to share their stories and seek the necessary support without fear of judgment.

Resources for Further Reading on Fibromyalgia Research

For those seeking to deepen their understanding of fibromyalgia, numerous resources are available. Organizations like the Fibromyalgia Foundation and the National Fibromyalgia Association provide valuable information, research updates, and support networks for individuals affected by the condition. These resources can help individuals connect with others who share similar experiences and gain insights into managing their symptoms.

Additionally, scientific journals and online databases offer access to the latest research findings on fibromyalgia. Staying informed about new developments can empower individuals to make informed decisions about their treatment and management strategies, fostering a proactive approach to living with fibromyalgia.

Personal Anecdotes from Individuals with Fibromyalgia

Personal anecdotes from individuals living with fibromyalgia can provide relatable insights and encouragement for those newly diagnosed. Sharing experiences can highlight the diversity of symptoms and coping strategies, demonstrating that there is no one-size-fits-all approach to managing the condition. These stories can also emphasize the importance of resilience and self-advocacy.

Listening to others' journeys can offer hope and practical tips for managing daily challenges. Many individuals share techniques that have helped them, such as mindfulness practices, gentle exercise, and dietary adjustments. These anecdotes can serve as a source of inspiration, encouraging others to explore different avenues for relief and support.

Inspirational Quotes to Motivate Readers

Inspirational quotes can serve as powerful reminders of strength and resilience for individuals coping with fibromyalgia. Phrases like "You are stronger than your struggles" or "Every day may not be good, but there is something good in every day" can uplift spirits and foster a positive mindset. These affirmations can encourage individuals to embrace their journey and focus on the progress made, rather than just the challenges faced.

Incorporating motivational quotes into daily routines, such as journaling or creating vision boards, can enhance mental well-being. Sharing these quotes within support groups can also build community and solidarity among those facing similar battles, reinforcing that they are not alone in their experiences.

CHAPTER 2:

Symptoms and Diagnosis

List of Common Symptoms of Fibromyalgia

Fibromyalgia is characterized by a range of symptoms that can significantly impact daily life. Common symptoms include widespread pain, fatigue, sleep disturbances, cognitive difficulties (often referred to as "fibro fog"), and increased sensitivity to pain. Other symptoms may involve headaches, irritable bowel syndrome (IBS), anxiety, and depression, leading to a multifaceted challenge for those affected. Understanding these symptoms is crucial for individuals as it sets the groundwork for recognizing the condition and seeking appropriate help.

To manage these symptoms effectively, individuals should note their experiences and how they affect their lives. This documentation can be invaluable for healthcare providers when diagnosing and creating a treatment plan. Keeping a symptom log can help in identifying patterns, triggers, and the severity of symptoms, allowing for tailored strategies to address the unique needs of the individual.

Explanation of How Symptoms May Vary Among Individuals

Fibromyalgia symptoms can manifest differently from person to person, making it a complex condition to understand and manage. Factors such as genetics, stress levels, co-existing conditions, and lifestyle choices can influence the severity and type of symptoms experienced. For instance, one individual may struggle primarily with fatigue, while another may find pain to be their dominant symptom.

Recognizing these variations is important for both individuals and healthcare providers to create effective management strategies. Personalized approaches to treatment are essential, as what works for one person may not be effective for another. Encouraging open communication about individual experiences helps in developing customized care plans that consider each person's unique symptom profile.

Overview of Diagnostic Criteria (e.g., ACR Criteria)

Diagnosing fibromyalgia often involves adhering to specific criteria established by the American College of Rheumatology (ACR). The ACR criteria include the presence of widespread pain lasting more than three months and the presence of additional symptoms such as fatigue, sleep disturbances, and cognitive dysfunction. Understanding these criteria can guide individuals in discussing their symptoms with healthcare professionals.

The criteria also emphasize the need for a comprehensive assessment of symptoms and their impact on daily functioning. Awareness of these diagnostic standards helps individuals articulate their experiences better and ensures they receive a thorough evaluation that considers all aspects of their condition.

Importance of a Comprehensive Medical History

A comprehensive medical history is crucial for diagnosing fibromyalgia and distinguishing it from other conditions with similar symptoms. Individuals should prepare a detailed account of their health history, including previous illnesses, family medical history, and any treatments or medications they have undergone. This information can assist healthcare providers in understanding the context of the symptoms and their potential causes.

Providing a thorough medical history allows for a more accurate diagnosis and can reveal patterns that might not be immediately apparent. It ensures that healthcare providers have all the necessary information to rule out other conditions and identify any potential underlying issues that could contribute to fibromyalgia symptoms.

Common Tests Used to Rule Out Other Conditions

Before diagnosing fibromyalgia, healthcare providers may conduct several tests to rule out other medical conditions that share similar symptoms. Common tests include blood tests, imaging studies (like X-rays or MRIs), and other specific assessments to check for inflammatory diseases, thyroid issues, or vitamin deficiencies. These tests help ensure that symptoms are not attributable to another underlying condition.

Understanding the purpose of these tests can alleviate anxiety for individuals undergoing diagnostic evaluations. It is essential for patients to engage with their healthcare providers about the testing process and to inquire about the relevance of each test to their symptoms.

Role of Symptom Journals in Diagnosis

Keeping a symptom journal is a practical strategy for individuals experiencing fibromyalgia symptoms. A symptom journal allows individuals to record their daily experiences, including the intensity of symptoms, activities, sleep patterns, and emotional well-being. This documentation can provide critical insights that help healthcare providers in diagnosing fibromyalgia and understanding individual triggers.

In addition to aiding diagnosis, a symptom journal can empower individuals to identify patterns over time. This awareness can assist in managing symptoms more effectively, allowing for the development of coping strategies tailored to specific triggers or situations.

The Significance of Tender Points in Diagnosis

Tender points are specific areas of the body that are sensitive to pressure in individuals with fibromyalgia.

Historically, the identification of 18 tender points was a key aspect of the ACR diagnostic criteria. Healthcare providers may apply pressure to these points during a physical examination to assess pain response, aiding in the diagnosis of fibromyalgia.

While tender points remain significant in diagnosis, the understanding of fibromyalgia has evolved, and healthcare providers now consider a broader range of symptoms and experiences. Recognizing tender points is still valuable but should be integrated into a comprehensive assessment that considers the individual's full symptom profile.

Diagnostic Challenges and Delays

Diagnosing fibromyalgia can be challenging and often involves a lengthy process. Many individuals experience delays in receiving a proper diagnosis due to the condition's complex and varied symptoms, which can overlap with other illnesses. Misdiagnosis is common, and some may face skepticism from healthcare providers unfamiliar with fibromyalgia.

To navigate these challenges, individuals should advocate for themselves, seeking second opinions or specialist referrals if necessary. Persistence and clear communication about symptoms are vital in ensuring that individuals receive the appropriate diagnosis and care.

Tips for Communicating Symptoms to Healthcare Providers

Effective communication with healthcare providers is essential for accurate diagnosis and treatment of fibromyalgia. Individuals should prepare for appointments by outlining their symptoms, noting their duration, intensity, and how they affect daily life. Being specific and providing examples can help convey the full scope of their experiences.

Additionally, individuals should feel empowered to ask questions about their symptoms and treatment options. Open dialogue fosters a collaborative relationship with healthcare providers, ensuring that concerns are addressed and that individuals feel heard and validated in their experiences.

Importance of Multidisciplinary Evaluation

A multidisciplinary evaluation is crucial for managing fibromyalgia, as the condition affects multiple aspects of health. This approach often involves various healthcare professionals, including primary care physicians, rheumatologists, physical therapists, and mental health specialists. Collaboration among these providers allows for a comprehensive understanding of the individual's condition and a more effective treatment plan.

Individuals should actively engage in their healthcare by seeking referrals to specialists and participating in a coordinated care approach. This holistic evaluation can address physical, emotional, and psychological aspects of fibromyalgia, leading to better outcomes and improved quality of life.

How to Prepare for a Doctor's Appointment

Preparing for a doctor's appointment can enhance the effectiveness of the visit, especially when dealing with fibromyalgia. Individuals should gather relevant medical records, a list of medications, and any notes on symptoms, including their frequency and triggers. This preparation ensures that healthcare providers have all necessary information to make informed decisions about diagnosis and treatment.

In addition to documenting symptoms, individuals should write down any questions or concerns they wish to address during the appointment. This proactive approach can facilitate more productive discussions and help ensure that individuals leave with a clearer understanding of their condition and the next steps in their care.

Understanding the Role of Specialists in Diagnosis

Specialists play a vital role in diagnosing and managing fibromyalgia, especially when symptoms are complex or resistant to initial treatment. Rheumatologists, neurologists, and pain specialists often have the expertise needed to conduct detailed evaluations and rule out other conditions. Their specialized knowledge allows for more tailored approaches to treatment and management.

Individuals should not hesitate to seek referrals to specialists when necessary. Understanding the role of these professionals in their healthcare journey can empower individuals to advocate for comprehensive evaluations that address all aspects of their fibromyalgia symptoms.

CHAPTER 3:

Causes and Triggers

Overview of Potential Causes of Fibromyalgia

Fibromyalgia is a complex condition characterized by widespread pain, fatigue, and various other symptoms. While the exact causes remain unclear, several factors are believed to contribute. These may include abnormalities in the way the brain processes pain signals, leading to heightened sensitivity to pain. Additionally, other conditions such as rheumatoid arthritis, lupus, and other autoimmune disorders can increase the likelihood of developing fibromyalgia.

Understanding the multifaceted nature of fibromyalgia is crucial for effective management. By acknowledging potential causes, individuals can better address their symptoms. This awareness allows for a more tailored approach to treatment, which may include medications, physical therapy, or lifestyle changes aimed at reducing overall pain and improving quality of life.

The Role of Genetics and Family History

Genetics play a significant role in the development of fibromyalgia. Research suggests that individuals with a family history of fibromyalgia or related conditions may have a higher risk of experiencing symptoms. This genetic predisposition can influence how the body responds to pain and stress, making some individuals more susceptible to developing the condition.

To understand your potential risk, consider discussing your family medical history with a healthcare provider. They can help identify if there are hereditary patterns and guide you in monitoring for symptoms, enabling earlier intervention and management strategies tailored to your unique situation.

Environmental Triggers That May Exacerbate Symptoms

Environmental factors can significantly impact the severity of fibromyalgia symptoms. Changes in weather, exposure to toxins, and even certain dietary choices can trigger flare-ups. For example, cold and damp weather may intensify pain, while prolonged exposure to stressors in the environment can lead to increased fatigue and discomfort.

To manage these triggers, individuals should be mindful of their surroundings and note any patterns associated with symptom exacerbation. Keeping a symptom diary can help identify specific environmental factors that worsen symptoms, allowing for proactive adjustments, such as avoiding certain climates or allergens.

Psychological Factors Contributing to Fibromyalgia

Psychological factors, including anxiety, depression, and stress, can play a crucial role in the development and exacerbation of fibromyalgia symptoms. These conditions can heighten the perception of pain and fatigue, creating a cycle that is difficult to break. Addressing mental health is therefore an essential component of managing fibromyalgia effectively.

Incorporating stress-reduction techniques, such as mindfulness, meditation, or cognitive behavioral therapy (CBT), can significantly improve symptoms. Engaging in regular mental health check-ins with a therapist can provide valuable tools and coping strategies, enhancing overall well-being.

How Trauma and Stress Impact Fibromyalgia

Trauma, whether physical or emotional, can serve as a catalyst for fibromyalgia. Research indicates that individuals with a history of traumatic experiences may have a heightened response to stress, which can trigger or worsen fibromyalgia symptoms. Understanding the connection between trauma and fibromyalgia can empower individuals to seek appropriate care and support.

To manage the effects of trauma, consider exploring therapies focused on trauma recovery, such as EMDR (Eye Movement Desensitization and Reprocessing) or somatic experiencing. These therapeutic approaches can help process trauma and reduce its impact on daily functioning, potentially alleviating fibromyalgia symptoms.

Lifestyle Factors That May Trigger Flare-Ups

Certain lifestyle choices can influence the frequency and intensity of fibromyalgia flare-ups. Poor diet, lack of exercise, and insufficient sleep can exacerbate symptoms and overall health. For instance, a diet high in processed foods and sugars may increase inflammation, leading to heightened pain and fatigue.

Making conscious lifestyle changes can lead to improved symptom management. Establishing a balanced diet rich in whole foods, engaging in regular physical activity tailored to your ability, and prioritizing good sleep hygiene can significantly reduce the likelihood of flare-ups and enhance overall quality of life.

Overview of Hormonal Influences

Hormonal fluctuations can significantly affect fibromyalgia symptoms. Changes in hormones, such as during menstrual cycles, pregnancy, or menopause, may trigger or worsen symptoms. For instance, many women report increased pain and fatigue during their menstrual periods due to hormonal changes that affect pain sensitivity.

To address hormonal influences, individuals may consider tracking their symptoms in relation to their hormonal cycles. This awareness can help in discussing treatment options with healthcare providers, who may suggest hormonal therapies or other strategies to alleviate symptoms during challenging times.

Discussion on Sleep Disturbances and Their Effects

Sleep disturbances are common among those with fibromyalgia and can exacerbate pain and fatigue. Many individuals report issues such as insomnia, restless leg syndrome, or sleep apnea, which disrupt restorative sleep. Poor sleep quality can create a vicious cycle, as inadequate rest can lead to increased sensitivity to pain.

Improving sleep hygiene is essential for managing fibromyalgia symptoms. Establishing a consistent sleep routine, creating a comfortable sleep environment, and limiting stimulants before bedtime can enhance sleep quality. Additionally, seeking treatment for underlying sleep disorders can significantly improve overall health and well-being.

Importance of Identifying Personal Triggers

Identifying personal triggers is a vital step in managing fibromyalgia. Triggers can vary greatly between individuals and may include specific activities, foods, or environmental factors. Recognizing these triggers enables individuals to avoid or modify their exposure to them, thereby reducing symptom flare-ups.

Keeping a detailed symptom journal can aid in tracking patterns related to triggers. This practice not only helps identify specific triggers but also allows for informed discussions with healthcare providers, leading to more personalized management strategies tailored to individual needs.

Strategies for Managing Known Triggers

Once personal triggers have been identified, developing effective management strategies is crucial for symptom relief. This may involve lifestyle modifications, such as adjusting physical activity levels, improving dietary habits, or implementing stress-reduction techniques. For instance, if certain foods are identified as triggers, replacing them with healthier alternatives can help mitigate symptoms.

Additionally, utilizing techniques such as pacing, which involves balancing activity and rest, can help manage energy levels and prevent overexertion. Engaging in regular low-impact exercises, such as walking or yoga, can promote overall well-being while respecting physical limitations.

The Role of Inflammation and Immune Response

Inflammation and immune response may play a role in the development and maintenance of fibromyalgia symptoms. Research suggests that individuals with fibromyalgia may have altered immune responses that contribute to pain and fatigue. Understanding the inflammatory processes involved can help in developing targeted treatment options.

Incorporating anti-inflammatory foods into the diet, such as fatty fish, nuts, and leafy greens, may help reduce inflammation levels. Furthermore, discussing anti-inflammatory medication options with a healthcare provider can provide additional support in managing symptoms effectively.

Ongoing Research into the Causes of Fibromyalgia

Ongoing research is critical in uncovering the complexities of fibromyalgia. Scientists are exploring various factors, including genetic, neurobiological, and environmental influences, to better understand how they contribute to the condition. This research aims to identify potential biomarkers for diagnosis and develop more effective treatment options.

Staying informed about the latest findings can empower individuals with fibromyalgia. Engaging in supportive communities or following reputable sources can provide valuable updates on emerging treatments and research breakthroughs, fostering hope and resilience in managing the condition.

Personal Stories Highlighting Individual Triggers

Personal stories from individuals living with fibromyalgia can provide invaluable insights into the diverse experiences and triggers associated with the condition. These narratives often highlight how seemingly minor lifestyle choices, environmental factors, or psychological influences can lead to significant symptom changes. Sharing these experiences fosters a sense of community and understanding.

Reading about others' journeys can also inspire practical strategies for managing triggers. Whether through online forums, support groups, or social media, connecting with others can offer both emotional support and practical advice, making the journey with fibromyalgia feel less isolating and more manageable.

CHAPTER 4:

Managing Symptoms

Overview of Self-Management Strategies

Self-management strategies empower individuals with fibromyalgia to take an active role in managing their symptoms. These strategies include identifying triggers, establishing routines, and employing various techniques to alleviate pain and fatigue. Understanding one's body and recognizing patterns can help patients develop personalized approaches that work best for them, creating a sense of control over their health.

To implement self-management, start by keeping a symptom diary that logs daily experiences, including pain levels, activities, and emotional states. This can help identify potential triggers, such as stress or certain foods, enabling more effective decision-making in managing symptoms. Regularly reviewing this diary can lead to actionable insights and adjustments in your approach to daily life.

Importance of Establishing a Daily Routine

A structured daily routine can significantly impact fibromyalgia symptoms by providing predictability and stability. Establishing consistent wake-up and sleep times, scheduled meals, and dedicated periods for relaxation can help minimize fatigue and increase energy levels throughout the day. This sense of structure also aids in balancing activity with rest, which is crucial for symptom management.

To create a daily routine, prioritize activities and commitments while allowing for flexibility. Start with a morning routine that includes light stretching or meditation to set a positive tone for the day. Incorporate scheduled breaks to recharge, ensuring that you avoid overexertion while still engaging in meaningful activities.

Techniques for Pain Management (e.g., Hot/Cold Therapy)

Hot and cold therapies are effective methods for managing fibromyalgia-related pain. Heat can soothe tight muscles and improve circulation, while cold therapy reduces inflammation and numbs sharp pain. Simple techniques include using heating pads, warm baths, or cold packs, applied to the affected areas for about 20 minutes at a time.

To integrate these therapies into your routine, experiment with different methods to discover what works best for you. Consider alternating between heat and cold applications to optimize relief. Consistently incorporating these techniques can make a significant difference in managing daily discomfort.

Role of Physical Activity in Symptom Relief

Physical activity is vital for individuals with fibromyalgia, as it can help reduce pain, improve mood, and increase energy levels. Low-impact exercises, such as walking, cycling, or swimming, can enhance mobility without exacerbating symptoms. Regular physical activity releases endorphins, which serve as natural pain relievers and mood enhancers.

To get started, aim for at least 30 minutes of gentle exercise most days of the week. Begin with short, manageable sessions, gradually increasing duration and intensity as tolerated. Listen to your body and adjust activities based on how you feel, ensuring that exercise remains a positive and beneficial aspect of your self-care routine.

Overview of Alternative Therapies (e.g., Acupuncture, Massage)

Alternative therapies can complement traditional treatments for fibromyalgia by providing additional symptom relief and improving overall well-being. Acupuncture involves inserting thin needles into specific points to stimulate the body's natural healing processes, while massage therapy focuses on relieving muscle tension and improving circulation. Both techniques can help alleviate pain and promote relaxation.

To explore alternative therapies, seek licensed practitioners in your area and discuss potential benefits and expectations. Many individuals find it helpful to combine these therapies with other self-management strategies for a holistic approach to fibromyalgia care. Always consult with your healthcare provider before starting any new treatment to ensure it fits into your overall health plan.

Dietary Changes and Their Impact on Symptoms

Dietary changes can significantly affect fibromyalgia symptoms, with certain foods potentially triggering or alleviating pain and fatigue. A balanced diet rich in whole foods, fruits, vegetables, lean proteins, and healthy fats can support overall health. Some individuals find that reducing processed foods, sugar, and gluten can lead to symptom improvement.

To implement dietary changes, consider keeping a food diary to track what you eat and how it impacts your symptoms. Focus on gradual changes rather than drastic overhauls, such as incorporating more whole foods or eliminating specific triggers. Consulting with a nutritionist familiar with fibromyalgia can provide tailored guidance to help you find the best dietary approach for your needs.

Stress Management Techniques (e.g., Mindfulness, Meditation)

Stress management is crucial for individuals with fibromyalgia, as stress can exacerbate symptoms. Techniques such as mindfulness and meditation can help cultivate a state of calm and reduce feelings of anxiety. Mindfulness encourages living in the moment and observing thoughts without judgment, while meditation promotes relaxation and mental clarity.

To practice mindfulness, set aside a few minutes each day to focus on your breathing or engage in guided meditation. Apps and online resources can provide structured practices to help you get started. Regular practice can improve emotional resilience, allowing you to better manage stress and its effects on your fibromyalgia symptoms.

The Importance of Sleep Hygiene

Sleep hygiene plays a vital role in managing fibromyalgia symptoms, as poor sleep can intensify pain and fatigue. Establishing a calming bedtime routine, such as dimming lights, reading, or practicing relaxation exercises, can signal your body that it's time to wind down. Aim for 7-9 hours of quality sleep each night to support overall health and well-being.

To improve sleep hygiene, create a sleep-friendly environment by keeping your bedroom dark, quiet, and cool. Limit screen time before bed and avoid caffeine and heavy meals in the evening. If sleep issues persist, consult with a healthcare provider for additional strategies and potential treatments tailored to your needs.

Role of Hydration in Managing Fibromyalgia

Staying well-hydrated is essential for individuals with fibromyalgia, as dehydration can worsen fatigue and discomfort. Drinking enough water supports overall bodily functions and can help alleviate symptoms. Aim for at least 8-10 cups of fluids daily, adjusting based on activity levels and climate.

To maintain hydration, carry a reusable water bottle and set reminders to drink throughout the day. Incorporating hydrating foods, such as fruits and vegetables, into your meals can also contribute to your fluid intake. Monitoring your hydration status can help ensure that you feel your best while managing fibromyalgia.

Incorporating Gentle Exercises (e.g., Yoga, Swimming)

Gentle exercises like yoga and swimming can greatly benefit individuals with fibromyalgia. These activities promote flexibility, reduce muscle tension, and enhance relaxation. Yoga, in particular, combines physical movement with mindfulness, making it a valuable tool for managing stress and pain.

To incorporate gentle exercises into your routine, start with short sessions of yoga or swimming, focusing on techniques that suit your fitness level. Look for local classes or online resources to guide your practice. Regular participation in these activities can lead to improved physical and emotional well-being over time.

Creating a Support Network for Symptom Management

Building a support network is essential for individuals with fibromyalgia, as connecting with others who understand the condition can provide emotional and practical assistance. This network can include friends, family, healthcare providers, and support groups, both in-person and online, that offer shared experiences and encouragement.

To create a support network, reach out to trusted individuals and share your experiences with fibromyalgia. Consider joining local or online support groups that focus on chronic pain or fibromyalgia for additional resources and community. Actively engaging in discussions can foster relationships that provide support and motivation in your journey toward symptom management.

Importance of Tracking Symptoms and Progress

Tracking symptoms and progress is a vital aspect of managing fibromyalgia, as it helps individuals identify patterns and evaluate the effectiveness of treatments. Maintaining a symptom journal can provide valuable insights into triggers, pain levels, and the impact of various strategies on overall well-being.

To effectively track your symptoms, record daily experiences, including pain levels, activities, and any changes in mood or energy. Regularly reviewing this information can help you communicate more effectively with healthcare providers and make informed decisions about your self-management strategies, ensuring you stay proactive in your care.

Tips for Setting Realistic Goals in Symptom Management

Setting realistic goals is crucial for effective symptom management in fibromyalgia. Goals should be specific, measurable, achievable, relevant, and time-bound (SMART). This approach helps individuals stay motivated and focused while also allowing for flexibility based on changing symptoms and circumstances.

To set realistic goals, start by identifying one or two key areas of focus, such as increasing physical activity or improving sleep hygiene. Break these goals into smaller, actionable steps, and celebrate progress along the way. Regularly reassess your goals and adjust them as needed, ensuring they remain aligned with your health journey.

CHAPTER 5:

Treatment Options

Overview of Conventional Medical Treatments

Conventional medical treatments for fibromyalgia primarily focus on alleviating symptoms and improving quality of life. These treatments often involve a combination of medications, physical therapy, and lifestyle changes. Physicians typically tailor these approaches based on individual patient needs and symptoms, ensuring that care are comprehensive and well-coordinated.

For effective management, it's crucial to work closely with healthcare providers to develop a personalized treatment plan. Regular assessments allow for adjustments to medications and therapies, addressing any new symptoms that may arise. Keeping an open line of communication with your healthcare team can lead to better outcomes and increased support throughout the treatment journey.

Common Medications Prescribed for Fibromyalgia

Several medications are commonly prescribed for managing fibromyalgia symptoms. These include pain relievers, antidepressants, and anti-seizure medications, which help reduce pain and improve sleep quality. Medications such as duloxetine (Cymbalta) and pregabalin (Lyrica) are often effective in alleviating fibromyalgia-related pain and fatigue.

It's important to discuss potential side effects and interactions with other medications with your doctor. They can help you find the right dosage and medication that works best for you, emphasizing the importance of patience and persistence in finding the most effective treatment regimen.

Non-Pharmacological Treatments (e.g., Cognitive-Behavioral Therapy)

Non-pharmacological treatments, such as cognitive-behavioral therapy (CBT), play a significant role in managing fibromyalgia. CBT helps patients identify and change negative thought patterns, which can contribute to pain perception and emotional distress. By learning coping strategies and relaxation techniques, individuals can improve their overall mental well-being and potentially reduce the severity of their symptoms.

Engaging in CBT often requires working with a trained therapist who specializes in chronic pain management. The process typically involves setting specific goals, practicing mindfulness, and applying new techniques in daily life, ultimately empowering patients to take control of their health and emotional responses to pain.

The Role of Physical Therapy in Treatment

Physical therapy is a vital component of fibromyalgia management, focusing on improving strength, flexibility, and overall physical function. A physical therapist can create a customized exercise program that includes low-impact aerobic exercises, stretching, and strength training, all aimed at reducing pain and increasing endurance.

Patients are encouraged to participate actively in their therapy sessions, gradually increasing activity levels based on their comfort and abilities. Consistency in attending physical therapy sessions, coupled with practicing recommended exercises at home, can significantly enhance physical health and reduce fibromyalgia symptoms over time.

Overview of Dietary Supplements and Their Benefits

Dietary supplements can be beneficial for individuals with fibromyalgia, as they may help alleviate symptoms and enhance overall wellness. Common supplements include omega-3 fatty acids, vitamin D, magnesium, and Coenzyme Q10, all of which may support pain relief and energy levels. Before starting any supplements, it's crucial to consult with a healthcare provider to ensure safety and effectiveness.

Incorporating these supplements into your daily routine can be straightforward. Many supplements are available in easy-to-swallow capsules or powders that can be mixed into smoothies or meals, making it easier to establish a consistent regimen for symptom relief.

Importance of Regular Follow-Ups with Healthcare Providers

Regular follow-ups with healthcare providers are essential for effective fibromyalgia management. These appointments allow for monitoring of symptoms, evaluation of treatment efficacy, and necessary adjustments to medication or therapy. Keeping a symptom diary can help track progress and provide valuable information during consultations.

To make the most of your appointments, prepare a list of questions and concerns ahead of time. This proactive approach enables patients to take an active role in their healthcare, fostering a collaborative relationship with their providers and ensuring comprehensive management of their condition.

Discussing Treatment Plans with Medical Professionals

Open communication about treatment plans with medical professionals is crucial in managing fibromyalgia. Patients should feel empowered to discuss their symptoms, treatment preferences, and any concerns they may have about prescribed therapies. This dialogue helps create a personalized approach that addresses individual needs and preferences.

When discussing treatment options, it's beneficial to ask questions about the benefits and potential side effects of each choice. Engaging in this collaborative decision-making process can lead to better adherence to treatment plans and improved health outcomes.

Integrating Holistic Approaches into Treatment Plans

Integrating holistic approaches into treatment plans can enhance overall well-being and symptom relief for individuals with fibromyalgia. Techniques such as acupuncture, yoga, meditation, and massage therapy can complement conventional treatments and provide additional benefits, such as reducing stress and improving relaxation.

To begin incorporating holistic approaches, start with one or two methods that resonate with you. Gradually explore additional options as you discover what works best for your body and mind, ensuring that these approaches align with your overall treatment strategy.

Navigating Insurance Coverage for Treatments

Navigating insurance coverage for fibromyalgia treatments can be challenging. Understanding your policy's specifics regarding medication, therapy, and alternative treatments is vital to avoid unexpected costs. Contacting your insurance provider for clarity on coverage limits and co-pays for different services can provide a clearer picture of your financial responsibilities.

When seeking treatment, keep detailed records of your healthcare expenses and any communication with your insurance provider. This documentation can help resolve disputes or clarify coverage issues, ensuring you receive the necessary support without financial strain.

Importance of Patient Education in Treatment Choices

Patient education is fundamental in making informed treatment choices for fibromyalgia. Understanding the condition, available treatments, and potential side effects empowers patients to participate actively in their care. Educational resources, such as books, workshops, and online forums, can provide valuable insights and help clarify misconceptions.

Patients should also seek to understand their own bodies and responses to various treatments. By staying informed about their condition and available options, individuals can make confident decisions that align with their health goals and preferences.

Success Stories from Individuals Exploring Different Treatments

Success stories from individuals who have explored various treatments for fibromyalgia can offer inspiration and insight. Many people find relief through a combination of traditional and alternative therapies, emphasizing the importance of personalizing treatment plans. These narratives highlight the diversity of approaches that can be taken, encouraging others to explore different options.

Listening to these experiences can provide practical ideas and motivation for those seeking symptom relief. Connecting with support groups or online communities can further foster a sense of belonging and shared understanding, creating a network of support as individuals navigate their own journeys.

Tips for Staying Informed About New Treatment Options

Staying informed about new treatment options for fibromyalgia is essential in managing this chronic condition. Patients can subscribe to reputable health newsletters, follow relevant medical organizations, and participate in online forums to receive the latest research updates and treatment recommendations.

Attending workshops or conferences can also provide valuable insights and networking opportunities with healthcare professionals and other patients. By actively seeking information and staying engaged with the fibromyalgia community, individuals can discover new therapies and strategies that may enhance their treatment experience.

Encouragement to Personalize Treatment Plans

Personalizing treatment plans is crucial in effectively managing fibromyalgia. Every individual's experience with the condition is unique, and treatment should reflect this diversity. Patients are encouraged to actively participate in their care by discussing preferences and experiences with their healthcare team to develop a plan tailored to their specific needs.

Trying different approaches and being open to adjustments is essential in finding the right combination of therapies. By focusing on what works best for their body and lifestyle, individuals can create a more effective and sustainable management plan that fosters a better quality of life.

CHAPTER 6:

Lifestyle Modifications

Importance of a Healthy Diet in Managing Symptoms

A balanced diet plays a crucial role in managing fibromyalgia symptoms, as certain foods can help reduce inflammation and promote overall health. Focus on consuming whole foods, such as fruits, vegetables, lean proteins, whole grains, and healthy fats. Avoid processed foods, excessive sugars, and trans fats, which can trigger inflammation and exacerbate symptoms.

To implement dietary changes, start by planning your meals around these healthy food groups. Preparing meals at home allows you to control ingredients and avoid hidden additives. Consider keeping a food diary to track what you eat and how it affects your symptoms, helping you identify any specific triggers.

Overview of Anti-Inflammatory Foods

Anti-inflammatory foods can be beneficial in managing fibromyalgia symptoms. Foods rich in omega-3 fatty acids, such as fatty fish, flaxseeds, and walnuts, can help reduce inflammation. Additionally, fruits and vegetables high in antioxidants, like berries and leafy greens, contribute to overall health and may alleviate pain.

Incorporate these foods into your diet by adding them to smoothies, salads, or as snacks. Experiment with spices such as turmeric and ginger, known for their anti-inflammatory properties, by adding them to soups, stews, or marinades for added flavor and health benefits.

Benefits of Regular Physical Activity for Fibromyalgia Patients

Engaging in regular physical activity can significantly improve symptoms of fibromyalgia, including pain, fatigue, and mood. Exercise releases endorphins, which act as natural pain relievers and can enhance your sense of well-being. Low-impact activities such as walking, swimming, or yoga are particularly effective and easier on the joints.

To start, aim for at least 30 minutes of moderate exercise most days of the week. Break it down into manageable sessions, such as three 10-minute walks, if needed. Consistency is key; find an activity you enjoy to help maintain motivation and make exercise a regular part of your routine.

Strategies for Incorporating Exercise into Daily Life

Incorporating exercise into daily life can be made easier with a few simple strategies. Start by setting realistic goals and creating a weekly schedule that includes time for physical activity. Consider activities that fit naturally into your day, such as walking during lunch breaks or using the stairs instead of the elevator.

Additionally, consider joining a group or finding a workout buddy to stay accountable and make exercise more enjoyable. Use reminders on your phone or calendar to keep you on track, and celebrate your achievements, no matter how small, to maintain motivation.

Importance of Sleep and Tips for Improving Sleep Quality

Quality sleep is vital for managing fibromyalgia symptoms, as poor sleep can worsen pain and fatigue. Establishing a regular sleep schedule, going to bed, and waking up at the same time each day can help regulate your body's internal clock. Create a relaxing bedtime routine to signal to your body that it's time to wind down.

To improve sleep quality, optimize your sleep environment by keeping your bedroom dark, cool, and quiet. Avoid caffeine and electronics before bed, as they can interfere with sleep. Consider relaxation techniques such as deep breathing or gentle stretches before sleep to help calm your mind and body.

Managing Stress Through Lifestyle Changes

Managing stress is essential for individuals with fibromyalgia, as stress can exacerbate symptoms. Implementing lifestyle changes such as time management, prioritizing tasks, and practicing relaxation techniques can help reduce stress levels. Identify stressors in your life and work on strategies to address or minimize them.

Incorporate activities that promote relaxation, such as meditation, yoga, or journaling, into your daily routine. Setting aside time for self-care activities and engaging in hobbies can also provide a much-needed break and help maintain a positive outlook.

The Impact of Social Support on Health Outcomes

Social support plays a crucial role in the well-being of individuals with fibromyalgia. Engaging with friends, family, or support groups can provide emotional comfort and practical advice for coping with symptoms. Sharing experiences with others who understand can help alleviate feelings of isolation.

To build a support network, reach out to loved ones or consider joining a local or online support group for people with fibromyalgia. Attend events or workshops focused on health and wellness, where you can meet others facing similar challenges and exchange coping strategies.

Tips for Setting Boundaries to Avoid Overexertion

Setting boundaries is vital in preventing overexertion and managing fibromyalgia symptoms. Learn to recognize your limits and communicate them clearly to others. Don't hesitate to say no to activities that you know will lead to excessive fatigue or stress.

Consider prioritizing tasks and focusing on what is essential, delegating when possible. Create a balance between activities and rest, scheduling downtime into your day to recharge. This approach allows you to engage in social or work activities while still taking care of your health.

Importance of Self-Care and Personal Time

Self-care is essential for managing fibromyalgia symptoms and maintaining mental health. Carve out time each day for activities that bring you joy and relaxation, whether it's reading, taking a bath, or spending time in nature. Prioritizing personal time helps rejuvenate your mind and body.

Incorporate self-care into your routine by setting aside specific time blocks for these activities. Treat them as appointments that you cannot miss. Encourage family and friends to support your self-care efforts, helping to ensure you have the time and space needed for personal well-being.

Role of Mindfulness Practices in Lifestyle Modification

Mindfulness practices, such as meditation and deep breathing, can help reduce stress and enhance your overall well-being. These techniques promote relaxation and can assist in managing fibromyalgia symptoms by increasing awareness of the present moment and reducing negative thought patterns.

To start practicing mindfulness, set aside a few minutes each day for meditation or deep breathing exercises. Consider guided sessions through apps or videos to help you stay focused. Regular practice can lead to improved emotional regulation and a greater sense of control over your symptoms.

Incorporating Creative Outlets and Hobbies

Engaging in creative activities and hobbies can be therapeutic for individuals with fibromyalgia. Creative outlets, such as painting, writing, or crafting, provide a means of self-expression and can help distract from pain. They also foster a sense of accomplishment, boosting your mood.

Make time for hobbies by scheduling them into your week. Explore different activities to find what resonates with you and keeps you engaged. Joining a local class or online community can also provide motivation and connect you with others who share similar interests.

Importance of Hydration and Its Effects on Symptoms

Staying hydrated is crucial for overall health and can positively affect fibromyalgia symptoms. Dehydration can lead to increased fatigue and muscle cramps, exacerbating pain. Aim to drink plenty of water throughout the day, and consider incorporating hydrating foods like cucumbers and watermelon into your diet.

To maintain hydration, keep a water bottle with you at all times and set reminders to drink water at regular intervals. Infusing water with fruits or herbs can make hydration more enjoyable. Monitoring your fluid intake can help ensure you stay adequately hydrated and support your body's functions.

Encouragement to Celebrate Small Victories in Lifestyle Changes

Celebrating small victories is important for maintaining motivation and fostering a positive mindset. Acknowledge your progress, no matter how minor, and take time to reflect on your accomplishments in managing fibromyalgia. This practice reinforces your efforts and encourages you to keep moving forward.

Consider keeping a journal to track your achievements and the positive changes you notice in your symptoms. Sharing your successes with friends or support groups can also enhance your sense of community and inspire others facing similar challenges.

CHAPTER 7:

Coping with Fatigue

Understanding Fatigue in Fibromyalgia Patients

Fatigue in fibromyalgia patients is a complex and multifaceted issue, often described as a debilitating sense of tiredness that affects daily functioning. It can stem from various factors, including disrupted sleep patterns, chronic pain, and psychological stress. Patients may find that their fatigue is disproportionate to their level of activity, leading to frustration and feelings of helplessness. Understanding this fatigue involves recognizing that it is not just physical tiredness but can also encompass mental and emotional exhaustion.

To address fatigue, it's essential for patients to track their symptoms and identify patterns related to their energy levels. Keeping a diary can help pinpoint times when fatigue worsens, allowing individuals to recognize potential triggers, whether they be stressors, overexertion, or even certain foods. This understanding lays the groundwork for more effective management strategies tailored to each individual's needs.

Strategies for Managing Fatigue Levels

Managing fatigue levels in fibromyalgia involves implementing practical strategies that promote energy conservation and enhance overall well-being. One effective approach is to prioritize tasks by focusing on essential activities and breaking larger tasks into smaller, manageable steps. Utilizing tools like timers or checklists can aid in keeping track of progress and help prevent overwhelming feelings.

Another strategy is to incorporate gentle physical activity, such as stretching or yoga, which can improve circulation and reduce muscle stiffness. Even short, low-intensity exercises can enhance energy levels without causing excessive fatigue. Establishing a routine that balances activity and rest is vital, allowing individuals to engage in movement while respecting their energy limitations.

Importance of Energy Conservation Techniques

Energy conservation techniques are crucial for fibromyalgia patients to maintain a balance between activity and rest. These techniques involve planning daily tasks in a way that minimizes fatigue and maximizes productivity. Simple changes, such as sitting while cooking or using assistive devices for household chores, can significantly reduce energy expenditure.

Additionally, patients can employ the "Pace Yourself" method by alternating periods of activity with rest breaks. This strategy allows individuals to engage in daily tasks without overexerting themselves, ultimately preventing exacerbation of fatigue. By being mindful of energy use, fibromyalgia patients can lead more fulfilling lives with improved functionality.

Creating a Balanced Daily Schedule

A balanced daily schedule is fundamental for managing fibromyalgia symptoms, particularly fatigue. By creating a structured routine, individuals can allocate time for activities, rest, and self-care, helping to regulate their energy levels throughout the day. A practical tip is to categorize tasks into "high energy" and "low energy" activities, allowing for better planning according to how one feel at different times.

Incorporating breaks and downtime into the schedule is equally important. Setting aside specific times for relaxation, hobbies, or light physical activities ensures that energy is replenished regularly. This thoughtful approach promotes a sense of control over daily life and helps to mitigate the unpredictable nature of fibromyalgia fatigue.

Role of Napping and Rest Periods

Napping and scheduled rest periods play a significant role in managing fatigue for fibromyalgia patients. Short naps of 20 to 30 minutes can provide a quick energy boost without disrupting nighttime sleep. Patients can benefit from listening to their bodies and taking naps when they feel fatigued, rather than waiting until they are completely drained.

In addition to napping, integrating rest periods throughout the day can prevent fatigue from building up. Patients should aim to take breaks during tasks, allowing time to relax and recharge. This practice not only reduces overall fatigue but also enhances productivity by making it easier to return to activities with renewed energy.

Importance of Mental Health Support for Fatigue Management

Mental health support is crucial for effective fatigue management in fibromyalgia patients, as emotional well-being directly influences energy levels. Therapy or counseling can help individuals process their feelings related to chronic fatigue, offering coping strategies to deal with frustration and emotional distress. Connecting with mental health professionals can provide valuable insights and techniques for managing anxiety and depression, which often accompany fibromyalgia.

Support groups, whether in-person or online, can also offer a sense of community and understanding. Sharing experiences and learning from others facing similar challenges can empower patients to develop resilience and foster positive mental health. By prioritizing mental health, individuals can create a more holistic approach to managing fatigue.

Coping Strategies for Mental Fatigue

Coping with mental fatigue involves employing specific strategies that target cognitive and emotional exhaustion. Mindfulness techniques, such as meditation or deep-breathing exercises, can help clear the mind and reduce stress levels. These practices promote relaxation and improve focus, making daily tasks feel more manageable.

Another effective coping strategy is engaging in enjoyable activities that stimulate the mind, such as reading or creative hobbies. Allocating time for these pursuits can provide mental breaks and a sense of accomplishment, which is beneficial for overall well-being. Finding balance between productivity and leisure can alleviate feelings of mental fatigue.

Identifying and Addressing Fatigue Triggers

Identifying fatigue triggers is essential for fibromyalgia patients to manage their symptoms effectively. Keeping a symptom diary can help individuals track their daily activities, sleep patterns, and emotional states, allowing them to pinpoint factors that lead to increased fatigue. This self-awareness empowers patients to make informed choices about their routines and lifestyles.

Once triggers are identified, addressing them becomes vital. This may involve adjusting schedules, reducing stressors, or implementing changes in diet and sleep hygiene. By actively managing these triggers, individuals can create a more balanced and sustainable approach to living with fibromyalgia.

Importance of Regular Check-Ins with Oneself

Regular self-check-ins are important for monitoring energy levels and overall well-being in fibromyalgia patients. Taking a few moments throughout the day to assess one's physical and emotional state can help identify when fatigue is becoming overwhelming. This practice encourages patients to listen to their bodies and make adjustments as needed, such as taking breaks or modifying activities.

Implementing self-check-ins can also foster greater self-awareness, helping individuals understand their limits and recognize early signs of fatigue. This proactive approach promotes a more mindful lifestyle, enabling patients to respond to their needs rather than react to fatigue after it occurs.

Discussion on the Role of Nutrition in Energy Levels

Nutrition plays a critical role in managing energy levels for fibromyalgia patients. Consuming a balanced diet rich in whole foods, such as fruits, vegetables, lean proteins, and whole grains, can help maintain stable energy levels throughout the day. It's essential to limit processed foods and sugars that can lead to energy crashes and exacerbate fatigue.

Incorporating small, frequent meals can also support energy levels by preventing dips in blood sugar. Patients should focus on nutrient-dense foods that provide sustained energy, like nuts, seeds, and legumes. By making mindful dietary choices, individuals can positively influence their energy levels and overall health.

Techniques for Staying Motivated Despite Fatigue

Staying motivated while dealing with fatigue can be challenging, but several techniques can help. Setting realistic goals and breaking them down into smaller, achievable tasks can create a sense of accomplishment without overwhelming oneself. Celebrating small victories can foster a positive mindset and encourage continued progress.

Another useful technique is to find sources of inspiration, such as motivational quotes or success stories from others with fibromyalgia. Surrounding oneself with supportive people and engaging in activities that bring joy can also help maintain motivation during difficult times. By focusing on positivity, individuals can combat feelings of fatigue and remain engaged in their lives.

Personal Stories on Managing Fatigue Successfully

Personal stories of managing fatigue successfully can provide valuable insights and encouragement for fibromyalgia patients. Hearing how others have navigated similar challenges can inspire hope and offer practical tips that resonate. Sharing experiences through support groups or online communities can create a sense of connection and understanding.

Individuals may find that strategies like pacing activities, prioritizing rest, and incorporating mindfulness have been effective for others. These shared experiences can validate feelings and provide new perspectives on managing fatigue, illustrating that recovery and improvement are possible through persistence and adaptation.

Encouragement to Seek Professional Help for Severe Fatigue

For those experiencing severe fatigue that interferes with daily life, seeking professional help is crucial. Healthcare providers can offer tailored advice, conduct necessary evaluations, and recommend treatment options that may include medication, therapy, or alternative therapies. It's important to address severe fatigue early to prevent it from significantly impacting quality of life.

Encouragement to consult with professionals can also come from support networks or online resources. Many individuals find that taking this step leads to improved management of their symptoms, allowing them to engage more fully in life. Professionals can provide the support and guidance needed to navigate the complexities of fibromyalgia and chronic fatigue.

CHAPTER 8:

Support Systems

Importance of Having a Support Network

Having a support network is essential for individuals managing fibromyalgia. A strong network provides emotional support; helps in coping with the chronic pain and fatigue associated with the condition, and can offer practical assistance in daily tasks. Connecting with others who understand your struggles can significantly alleviate feelings of isolation and enhance overall well-being.

To build a support network, identify individuals in your life who can be supportive, whether they are family members, friends, or peers. Engaging in local or online communities can also be beneficial, as they provide spaces to share experiences and strategies for managing fibromyalgia, creating a sense of belonging and mutual understanding.

Different Types of Support (Family, Friends, Online Communities)

Support for fibromyalgia can come from various sources, including family, friends, and online communities. Family and friends can provide immediate emotional and physical support, while online communities offer a broader network of people who share similar experiences. These connections can help you feel less alone and provide a wealth of information and encouragement.

To tap into these different types of support, maintain open lines of communication with loved ones about your needs and challenges. Explore online forums, social media groups, or local support groups specifically focused on fibromyalgia to connect with others who understand the unique challenges you face.

How to Communicate Needs to Family and Friends

Effectively communicating your needs to family and friends is crucial in managing fibromyalgia. Start by explaining your condition in simple terms, highlighting how it affects your daily life and the specific types of support you require. Use clear examples, such as needing help with household chores or wanting companionship during doctor visits, to illustrate your needs.

Additionally, encourage open dialogue by inviting questions and offering to share resources about fibromyalgia. This helps your loved ones understand your situation better and fosters an environment where they feel comfortable discussing their own concerns and feelings.

Overview of Fibromyalgia Support Groups

Fibromyalgia support groups provide a safe space for individuals to share experiences, coping strategies, and emotional support. These groups often meet in person or online and can be facilitated by healthcare professionals or peer-led. Participating in these groups can help reduce feelings of isolation and increase understanding of the condition through shared experiences.

To find a support group, consider searching online platforms, local community centers, or hospitals that may host these gatherings. Joining a group can empower you to connect with others who are navigating similar challenges, fostering a sense of community and shared resilience.

Role of Therapists and Counselors in Support

Therapists and counselors play a vital role in supporting individuals with fibromyalgia. They provide a professional perspective on coping mechanisms and emotional support strategies. Therapy can help address the emotional toll of living with chronic pain and fatigue, offering tools to manage stress, anxiety, and depression that may accompany fibromyalgia.

To benefit from therapy, seek out professionals experienced in chronic pain management or fibromyalgia. Regular sessions can help you develop personalized strategies for coping with symptoms, enhancing your overall quality of life and providing a safe space to express your feelings and concerns.

Importance of Sharing Experiences with Others

Sharing your experiences with fibromyalgia can be therapeutic and beneficial for both you and those around you. It fosters understanding, reduces stigma, and can create deeper connections with others who may be going through similar challenges. Expressing your journey can also empower you to advocate for yourself and raise awareness about the condition.

Consider writing a blog, participating in support groups, or simply talking with friends and family about your experiences. By sharing your story, you can inspire others to do the same, creating a community of support and understanding that is essential for coping with fibromyalgia.

Navigating Relationships with Fibromyalgia

Navigating relationships while managing fibromyalgia can be challenging. Chronic pain and fatigue can affect your ability to engage fully, leading to misunderstandings with loved ones. It's important to communicate openly about your condition, ensuring your friends and family understand that your limitations are not a reflection of your feelings towards them.

To maintain healthy relationships, set realistic expectations about your availability and energy levels. Encourage loved ones to ask questions and share their feelings about your condition, fostering a supportive environment where both parties can express their needs and concerns.

Resources for Finding Local and Online Support

Finding local and online resources for fibromyalgia support is crucial for building a strong support network. Local resources may include community health centers, hospitals, and libraries that host support groups or educational events. Online resources, such as forums, social media groups, and websites dedicated to fibromyalgia, can also provide valuable connections and information.

Start by searching online for fibromyalgia support groups or organizations in your area. Additionally, consider reaching out to healthcare providers for recommendations on local resources and support networks tailored to your needs.

Importance of Educating Loved Ones about Fibromyalgia

Educating your loved ones about fibromyalgia is vital for fostering understanding and support. By sharing information about the condition, its symptoms, and its impact on your daily life, you can help family and friends comprehend the challenges you face. This understanding can lead to more empathetic responses and better support in times of need.

To educate others, provide them with resources, such as articles, brochures, or books about fibromyalgia. Consider having open conversations to discuss what they can do to support you effectively, helping them understand how your experiences may differ from their own.

Tips for Maintaining Social Connections

Maintaining social connections while managing fibromyalgia can be difficult, but it's essential for emotional well-being. Prioritize quality over quantity by focusing on relationships that bring you joy and support. Schedule regular catch-ups with close friends and family, even if it's through a phone call or video chat, to maintain those bonds

Set realistic goals for social interactions based on your energy levels. Don't hesitate to decline invitations when you're feeling fatigued; instead, suggest alternative activities that accommodate your needs, such as a low-key gathering or a quiet day at home.

Personal Stories of Support Systems in Action

Personal stories of support systems can provide inspiration and hope for those dealing with fibromyalgia. Hearing how others have navigated their journey with support from family, friends, or community groups can highlight the importance of connection and resilience. These stories often illustrate practical strategies for building a supportive environment.

Consider sharing your own story or seeking out testimonials from others in similar situations. Engaging in these narratives can create a sense of solidarity and encourage individuals to cultivate their support networks, fostering a community of understanding and strength.

Strategies for Helping Others Understand Fibromyalgia

Helping others understand fibromyalgia involves sharing clear, accessible information about the condition and its effects. Use simple language to explain how fibromyalgia impacts your life and the specific challenges you face, such as fatigue, pain, and cognitive issues. Providing relatable examples can help them grasp the complexities of living with the condition.

Encourage open communication and be patient with their questions or misconceptions. Utilize resources, such as pamphlets or websites, to supplement your explanations, allowing loved ones to learn at their own pace and fostering a more supportive environment.

Importance of Self-Advocacy in Support Systems

Self-advocacy is crucial for navigating support systems when living with fibromyalgia. It involves clearly expressing your needs, preferences, and rights regarding your care and support. Advocating for yourself empowers you to take control of your situation and ensures that your voice is heard in conversations with healthcare providers, family, and friends.

To practice self-advocacy, start by identifying your needs and the areas where you require support. Use assertive communication techniques to express these needs, whether in person or through written correspondence.

CHAPTER 9:

Living Well with Fibromyalgia

Overview of Living a Fulfilling Life despite Fibromyalgia

Living with fibromyalgia can be challenging, but it's important to recognize that a fulfilling life is possible. Embracing a holistic approach that combines physical, emotional, and social well-being is crucial. This includes understanding your body's limits, prioritizing self-care, and integrating activities that bring joy and satisfaction into your daily routine. Finding hobbies and interests that align with your energy levels can help maintain a sense of normalcy and purpose.

Moreover, establishing a supportive network of friends, family, or online communities can greatly enhance your quality of life. Sharing experiences and coping strategies with others who understand your journey can foster connection and reduce feelings of isolation. Utilizing resources such as support groups or therapy can provide additional encouragement and tools for managing your condition.

Strategies for Setting Realistic Goals and Aspirations

Setting realistic goals is vital for maintaining motivation and a sense of achievement while living with fibromyalgia. Begin by identifying short-term goals that are attainable and measurable, such as incorporating a daily walk into your routine or dedicating time to a creative hobby. Break larger aspirations into smaller, manageable steps, allowing yourself to celebrate each achievement, no matter how small.

When setting these goals, it's essential to consider your current energy levels and any fluctuations you may experience. Keeping a journal to track your progress and adjust your goals accordingly can help ensure they remain realistic. This practice fosters a positive mindset, as you can visually see how far you've come, even on challenging days.

Importance of Staying Positive and Motivated

Maintaining a positive attitude can significantly impact your experience with fibromyalgia. One effective strategy is to practice gratitude by regularly reflecting on the aspects of your life that bring you joy or comfort. This can involve keeping a gratitude journal, where you note three things each day that you are thankful for, helping shift focus away from pain and fatigue.

Staying motivated often requires finding inspiration in your daily life. Engaging in activities that uplift your spirits—such as listening to music, practicing mindfulness, or connecting with loved ones—can provide moments of joy amidst the challenges. Additionally, surrounding yourself with supportive and positive individuals can reinforce a hopeful mindset.

Discussing Long-Term Management Plans

Creating a long-term management plan for fibromyalgia involves a comprehensive approach tailored to your unique needs. This may include a combination of medication, physical therapy, lifestyle changes, and alternative therapies such as acupuncture or yoga. Collaborating with healthcare professionals to develop a personalized plan can empower you to take control of your symptoms.

Regularly reviewing and adjusting your management plan is essential, as fibromyalgia symptoms can fluctuate. Keeping an open line of communication with your healthcare team and being proactive about reporting changes in your condition can help optimize your treatment strategy and improve your overall quality of life.

Overview of Successful Coping Strategies

Effective coping strategies for managing fibromyalgia symptoms can vary widely from person to person. Techniques such as mindfulness meditation, gentle exercise, and cognitive-behavioral therapy (CBT) have been shown to help many individuals cope with chronic pain and fatigue. Incorporating these practices into your daily routine can enhance your resilience against symptoms and promote emotional well-being.

Additionally, establishing a consistent sleep schedule and prioritizing rest is crucial for managing fatigue. Creating a calming bedtime routine can improve sleep quality, making you feel more energized and better equipped to handle daily challenges. Remember that finding the right coping strategies may take time, and it's important to remain patient and adaptable.

Role of Personal Stories in Inspiring Others

Personal stories can serve as powerful sources of inspiration for those living with fibromyalgia. Sharing your journey, including challenges and triumphs, can resonate with others facing similar struggles and foster a sense of community. Writing a blog, participating in support groups, or using social media to share your experiences can help create connections and provide encouragement.

Listening to the stories of others can also be enlightening, as it may offer new coping strategies or insights into living with fibromyalgia. By exchanging narratives, you contribute to a culture of support and understanding, reminding everyone that they are not alone in their experiences.

Importance of Celebrating Progress and Milestones

Recognizing and celebrating progress is essential in maintaining motivation and a positive mindset while living with fibromyalgia. Regularly taking time to acknowledge milestones—no matter how small—can reinforce a sense of achievement and resilience. This may involve treating yourself to something special or reflecting on how far you've come since your diagnosis.

Additionally, sharing your milestones with supportive friends and family can enhance this celebration. Encouragement from loved ones can amplify your sense of accomplishment and serve as a reminder of the positive strides you're making, even on difficult days.

Tips for Maintaining a Hopeful Outlook

Maintaining a hopeful outlook is key to navigating life with fibromyalgia. One effective strategy is to establish a daily routine that includes activities that uplift your spirit, such as engaging in hobbies, practicing gratitude, or enjoying nature. Taking time each day for self-care activities can help reinforce a positive mindset and improve your overall mood.

Connecting with others who share similar experiences can also foster hope. Engaging in support groups or online forums allows you to share challenges, victories, and coping strategies, creating a network of support that uplifts and motivates. This sense of community can be invaluable in maintaining hope and positivity in your journey.

Resources for Ongoing Education About Fibromyalgia

Staying informed about fibromyalgia is essential for effective management of the condition. Numerous resources are available, including reputable websites, books, and online courses dedicated to educating individuals about fibromyalgia, its symptoms, and management strategies. These resources can help you better understand your condition and explore new approaches to treatment.

Participating in webinars or local workshops can also provide valuable insights and connect you with experts in the field. Regularly engaging with updated information can empower you to make informed decisions about your health and explore new coping strategies that may enhance your quality of life.

The Significance of Resilience and Adaptability

Resilience and adaptability are critical qualities when navigating life with fibromyalgia. Embracing the unpredictability of your symptoms and learning to adjust your plans and expectations can significantly enhance your emotional well-being. Developing a flexible mindset allows you to respond positively to challenges and setbacks, fostering a sense of control over your life.

Building resilience can involve practicing self-compassion and recognizing that it's okay to have bad days. By accepting your limitations and adapting your goals accordingly, you can cultivate a more forgiving attitude towards yourself, which can ultimately improve your overall quality of life.

Personal Reflections on Living Well with Fibromyalgia

Reflecting on your personal journey with fibromyalgia can be a powerful tool for growth and understanding. Taking time to journal about your experiences, emotions, and coping mechanisms can help clarify what works best for you and how you've overcome obstacles. This practice not only enhances self-awareness but can also reveal patterns and strategies that contribute to your well-being.

Sharing these reflections with others, whether through a blog, support group, or personal conversations, can provide insight and encouragement. Your experiences may resonate with someone else, creating a ripple effect of support and hope within the fibromyalgia community.

Encouragement to Keep Pushing Forward

Continuing to push forward despite the challenges of fibromyalgia is essential for maintaining a fulfilling life. Cultivating a mindset of persistence involves focusing on small victories and reminding yourself that progress may come in different forms. Surrounding yourself with supportive individuals who encourage you during tough times can reinforce your determination and help you stay focused on your goals.

Moreover, engaging in regular self-reflection can help you identify your strengths and the resources available to you. Acknowledging your resilience in facing obstacles can inspire you to keep moving forward, reinforcing the belief that you are capable of overcoming challenges and living well with fibromyalgia.

Final Thoughts on Embracing Life with Fibromyalgia

Embracing life with fibromyalgia involves recognizing that while challenges exist, they do not define your entire experience. It's essential to focus on the aspects of life that bring joy, connection, and fulfillment. Developing a proactive approach to managing your symptoms and seeking out supportive communities can make a significant difference in your overall well-being.

Ultimately, living well with fibromyalgia is about finding balance, nurturing positivity, and celebrating the unique journey you're on. Embracing your strengths, sharing your story, and remaining open to new coping strategies can empower you to thrive despite the obstacles.

Common Concerns

Is Fibromyalgia a Real Condition?

Fibromyalgia is indeed a real and recognized medical condition characterized by widespread chronic pain, fatigue, and various other symptoms. It is classified as a syndrome rather than a disease, meaning it is a collection of symptoms that can affect individuals differently. The underlying causes are not entirely understood, but it is believed to involve a combination of genetic, environmental, and psychological factors that impact how the brain processes pain signals.

To validate its reality, medical professionals often rely on diagnostic criteria established by organizations such as the American College of Rheumatology. Symptoms include tenderness in specific areas, sleep disturbances, and cognitive difficulties, known as "fibro fog." Despite some misconceptions, extensive research and patient experiences affirm fibromyalgia's legitimacy as a complex condition.

How Long Does It Take to Get Diagnosed?

The diagnosis of fibromyalgia can take considerable time due to its complex nature and symptom overlap with other conditions. On average, patients may wait anywhere from three to five years to receive a definitive diagnosis. This delay often stems from the need for thorough evaluations to rule out other potential medical issues that might present similar symptoms, such as rheumatoid arthritis or chronic fatigue syndrome.

To facilitate diagnosis, it's essential to maintain a detailed symptom diary documenting pain levels, fatigue episodes, and other relevant experiences. This log can help healthcare providers identify patterns and determine if the symptoms align with fibromyalgia diagnostic criteria, streamlining the diagnostic process.

Can Fibromyalgia Symptoms Improve Over Time?

Fibromyalgia symptoms can vary significantly over time, with some individuals experiencing periods of remission or reduced severity. Factors such as lifestyle changes, effective management strategies, and appropriate treatments can contribute to symptom improvement. Regular monitoring and adjustments to treatment plans are crucial, as what works well initially may need to be modified as the condition evolves.

Engaging in a balanced routine that includes stress management techniques, physical activity, and healthy eating can enhance overall well-being. Patients are encouraged to communicate openly with their healthcare providers about any changes in symptoms, allowing for proactive adjustments to their management strategies.

What Are the Best Treatment Options?

The best treatment options for fibromyalgia typically involve a multi-faceted approach, combining medication, physical therapy, and lifestyle modifications. Common medications include pain relievers, antidepressants, and anticonvulsants, which help manage symptoms and improve quality of life. It is essential to work closely with a healthcare provider to determine the most effective medication regimen tailored to individual needs.

In addition to medications, non-pharmacological approaches such as cognitive-behavioral therapy, mindfulness techniques, and physical therapy can provide significant relief. Patients should consider incorporating complementary therapies, such as acupuncture or massage, into their treatment plans, as these can enhance symptom management and promote relaxation.

Is There a Cure for Fibromyalgia?

Currently, there is no known cure for fibromyalgia. However, effective management strategies can significantly reduce symptoms and improve quality of life for many individuals. Research continues to explore various treatment options, but the focus remains on symptom relief and functional improvement rather than a cure.

Patients should adopt a proactive approach to managing their condition by exploring different treatment avenues and customizing their management plans. Open communication with healthcare providers and a willingness to try various therapies can lead to significant symptom relief and improved overall well-being.

How Do I Manage Flare-Ups?

Managing flare-ups involves implementing strategies to reduce the severity and duration of symptoms during exacerbations. First, it is essential to identify potential triggers, such as stress, physical activity, or dietary changes, to help prevent future flare-ups. Keeping a journal can assist in tracking these triggers and recognizing patterns over time.

When a flare-up occurs, prioritizing self-care is crucial. Techniques such as applying heat or cold packs, engaging in gentle stretching or yoga, and ensuring adequate rest can provide relief. Additionally, practicing relaxation techniques, like deep breathing or meditation, can help reduce stress and manage flare-up symptoms more effectively.

Can Diet Affect My Fibromyalgia Symptoms?

Yes, diet can significantly impact fibromyalgia symptoms. Certain foods may exacerbate inflammation and contribute to pain and fatigue, while others can promote healing and alleviate symptoms. Patients are encouraged to adopt a balanced, anti-inflammatory diet that includes plenty of fruits, vegetables, whole grains, and healthy fats while minimizing processed foods and sugar.

Keeping a food diary can help identify any dietary triggers that may worsen symptoms. Patients should consider working with a registered dietitian familiar with fibromyalgia to develop personalized meal plans that cater to their individual needs and preferences.

How Can I Explain Fibromyalgia to Others?

Explaining fibromyalgia to others can be challenging due to misconceptions surrounding the condition. It's helpful to start with a brief description of fibromyalgia as a chronic disorder characterized by widespread pain, fatigue, and other symptoms that can significantly impact daily life. Emphasize that it is a real medical condition and not simply "in the head."

Providing resources, such as pamphlets or websites dedicated to fibromyalgia, can also aid in education. Encouraging open dialogue and sharing personal experiences can foster understanding and support from friends and family, making it easier to communicate the challenges of living with fibromyalgia.

What Role Does Exercise Play in Managing Symptoms?

Exercise plays a vital role in managing fibromyalgia symptoms by promoting overall health, reducing pain, and improving energy levels. Low-impact activities such as walking, swimming, or yoga are often recommended as they can help build strength and flexibility without exacerbating pain. It's essential to start slowly and gradually increase intensity based on individual tolerance.

Consistency is key; aim for regular exercise sessions several times a week. Incorporating stretching and relaxation techniques can further enhance the benefits of exercise, helping to manage stress and improve sleep quality, which is often disrupted in individuals with fibromyalgia.

Are There Support Groups for People with Fibromyalgia?

Yes, there are numerous support groups available for individuals with fibromyalgia, both online and in-person. These groups provide a safe space for individuals to share experiences, exchange coping strategies, and offer emotional support. Connecting with others who understand the challenges of living with fibromyalgia can alleviate feelings of isolation and provide valuable insights into effective management techniques.

To find a support group, consider reaching out to local healthcare providers or searching online forums and social media platforms. Many organizations dedicated to fibromyalgia offer resources and connections to support networks, making it easier to find the right group for individual needs.

How Can I Cope with Fatigue?

Coping with fatigue requires a multifaceted approach that includes lifestyle adjustments and self-care strategies. Prioritizing good sleep hygiene is crucial; establish a regular sleep schedule, create a restful environment, and avoid stimulants before bedtime to improve sleep quality. Incorporating short naps or rest periods during the day can also help manage fatigue levels.

Energy management techniques, such as pacing activities and breaking tasks into smaller, manageable steps, can be beneficial. Learning to recognize personal limits and asking for help when needed can prevent overexertion, allowing individuals to conserve energy and better cope with fatigue.

Can Mental Health Impact My Fibromyalgia?

Yes, mental health can significantly influence fibromyalgia symptoms. Stress, anxiety, and depression may exacerbate pain and fatigue, creating a cycle that can be difficult to break. It is essential to address mental health concerns alongside physical symptoms, as managing one can positively impact the other.

Incorporating mental health strategies such as counseling, cognitive-behavioral therapy, and mindfulness practices can help individuals cope with the emotional aspects of fibromyalgia. Establishing a supportive social network and practicing self-care can also improve mental health and, in turn, help manage fibromyalgia symptoms more effectively.

What Should I Do If I Feel Overwhelmed?

Feeling overwhelmed is common among individuals with fibromyalgia due to the constant challenges of managing symptoms. When overwhelmed, it's essential to take a step back and practice grounding techniques, such as deep breathing exercises or mindfulness meditation, to regain a sense of calm and clarity. Allow yourself to pause and acknowledge your feelings without judgment.

Additionally, creating a manageable to-do list can help prioritize tasks, breaking them down into smaller, more achievable steps. Don't hesitate to reach out for support from friends, family, or a therapist to share your feelings and gain perspective, making it easier to navigate overwhelming situations.

FAQs

Can fibromyalgia go into remission?

Fibromyalgia can fluctuate significantly from person to person. Some individuals report periods where their symptoms diminish, leading to what is often referred to as remission. This can be influenced by various factors, including lifestyle changes, treatment effectiveness, and overall health improvements. However, for many, fibromyalgia remains a chronic condition that may require ongoing management to maintain a better quality of life.

To work towards remission, it's essential to focus on symptom management strategies that suit your personal experience. Engaging in consistent physical activity, adhering to a balanced diet, and exploring relaxation techniques like yoga or meditation can all contribute positively. Keeping track of your symptoms and their triggers may also help you and your healthcare provider identify patterns that support your journey toward symptom reduction.

How can I get my doctor to take my symptoms seriously?

Communicating effectively with your healthcare provider is crucial for receiving the attention you need. Start by maintaining a detailed symptom diary where you document your daily experiences, including the intensity and duration of symptoms, activities that trigger pain, and any other relevant health changes. This diary serves as a valuable tool during appointments, helping you present clear and specific information that can facilitate a better understanding of your condition.

When discussing your symptoms, express your concerns openly and assertively. Make sure to explain how these symptoms impact your daily life, from work and social activities to mental health. A collaborative approach will help your doctor appreciate the seriousness of your situation, leading to a more tailored treatment plan.

What lifestyle changes can help manage fibromyalgia?

Implementing lifestyle changes can play a significant role in managing fibromyalgia symptoms. Regular exercise is often recommended, as low-impact activities like walking, swimming, or cycling can improve energy levels, reduce pain, and enhance mood. Aim for at least 30 minutes of moderate exercise most days of the week, gradually increasing intensity as tolerated. Pairing exercise with stretching or flexibility routines can further alleviate muscle stiffness.

In addition to physical activity, focusing on a balanced diet is essential. Incorporate whole foods, plenty of fruits and vegetables, and stay hydrated. Practicing stress management techniques such as mindfulness, deep breathing exercises, or yoga can also help improve overall well-being and reduce symptom flare-ups. Small, consistent changes in your daily routine can lead to substantial improvements in managing fibromyalgia.

Are there specific diets that help with fibromyalgia?

While there is no universally effective diet for fibromyalgia, certain dietary approaches can help manage symptoms. Many patients find that incorporating anti-inflammatory foods—such as fatty fish, nuts, seeds, fruits, and vegetables—can lead to noticeable improvements in their symptoms. Avoiding processed foods, added sugars, and trans fats is also recommended, as these can contribute to inflammation and worsen symptoms.

Experimenting with elimination diets may also be beneficial for identifying specific food triggers. Consider working with a healthcare provider or nutritionist to design a personalized eating plan. Keeping a food diary can help you track your intake and symptoms, making it easier to pinpoint which foods positively or negatively affect your health.

Can stress really worsen my symptoms?

Yes, stress is a significant trigger for fibromyalgia flare-ups. The body's stress response can lead to increased muscle tension and pain sensitivity, exacerbating symptoms. Understanding your stressors and implementing coping strategies is essential for managing fibromyalgia effectively. Techniques like deep breathing exercises, progressive muscle relaxation, or engaging in hobbies can help reduce stress levels and promote relaxation.

Additionally, consider establishing a daily routine that incorporates stress management practices. This could include setting aside time for relaxation, ensuring sufficient sleep, and participating in regular physical activity. Cultivating a support system of friends, family, or support groups can also alleviate feelings of isolation and provide encouragement in managing stress effectively.

Conclusion

Living with fibromyalgia can be challenging, but understanding the condition and adopting effective management strategies can significantly improve quality of life. This guide serves as a comprehensive resource for individuals navigating their fibromyalgia journey, offering insights, support, and practical solutions for symptom relief. By taking an active role in their health, readers can empower themselves to live well and thrive despite the challenges fibromyalgia presents.